Chancelier CIRIMWAMI

The bottleneck in the reorganization of the drug sector

Chancelier CIRIMWAMI

The bottleneck in the reorganization of the drug sector

An approach that requires involvement, ownership and redress by the political-administrative authorities

ScienciaScripts

Imprint

Cover image: www.ingimage.com

This book is a translation from the original published under ISBN 978-620-6-70867-4.

Publisher:
Sciencia Scripts
is a trademark of
Dodo Books Indian Ocean Ltd. and OmniScriptum S.R.L publishing group

120 High Road, East Finchley, London, N2 9ED, United Kingdom
Str. Armeneasca 28/1, office 1, Chisinau MD-2012, Republic of Moldova, Europe
Printed at: see last page
ISBN: 978-620-8-12095-5

TABLE OF CONTENTS

EPIGRAPH

According to Fayol, managing "means anticipating, organizing, controlling, coordinating and commanding".

ACKNOWLEDGEMENTS

We cannot claim exclusive ownership of this work, although most of it is our own. We give thanks to GOD our Creator and would like to take this opportunity to express our gratitude to all those who contributed to this study, for their commitment and availability throughout all phases.

This research would not have been as successful, or as complete, without the experimental input of the various participants, respectively my thesis director Emeritus Professor Bernard Gangloff and co-director Anne Marie Costalat Founeau, and the judicious advice of the late Professor Christian MUGISHO KATENGURA and the late Professor Daniel KAISHUSHA MBONYI.

To all these people and to all those who contributed to the writing of this work, we express our thanks.

ACRONYMS

ANSM	Agence Nationale de Sécurité du Médicament
BCZS	Health Zone Central Office
CDR	Regional Drug Distribution Center
CMM	Average monthly consumption
CT	Head of works
DC	: Order lead times
DCI	International Nonproprietary Name
DL	: Delivery times
DPM	Department of Pharmacy and Medicines
ECZS	Health Zone Management Team
FOSA	: Sanitary training
GIS	Management of healthcare institutions
HGR	General referral hospital
LNME	National List of Essential Medicines
MAD	Month of supply available
MCZS	Chief Medical Officer
MNU	Unused medication
WHO	World Health Organization
NGO	Non-governmental organization
UN	United Nations
PNAM	National Drug Supply Program

UNDP	United Nations Development Programme
SD	Available stock
SNA M	National Supply System
SRSS	Health Care Reinforcement System
SSP	: Primary Health Care
EU	European Union
ULGL	Université Libre des Grands Lacs
ZS	Health Zone
$	: Dollars
€	: Euro

SUMMARY

In view of the worrying situation regarding resistance to antibacterial drugs, a study was carried out on pharmacies that are not open to the public in Bukavu, in order to identify the factors that contribute to the emergence of resistance.

Our study aims to describe and analyze the management of medicines and medical consumables in pharmaceutical dispensaries open to the public in the Ibanda health zone, in order to determine the factors that negatively influence the dispensing of care and service within the facilities, and to propose recommendations.

As part of the national policy to improve the efficiency and viability of health structures, several efforts are being made, but the results remain mixed. The case of pharmaceutical dispensaries open to the public in the Ibanda health zone is marked by the poor provision of health services in these structures. Documentary analysis, observation and interviews with pharmaceutical service providers enabled us to determine efficiency and viability, and to describe the process for managing medicines and medical consumables in pharmacies open to the public.

Our analyses show that in the pharmaceutical dispensaries open to the public in the Ibanda health zone, people directly involved in the management of medicines and medical consumables within :

- *Most of the respondents are women, who work more in pharmaceutical dispensaries, and the 25 to 49 age bracket is in the majority, with a median age of 27, and most have a university education;*
- *Most pharmaceutical service providers have a low proportion of pharmacy science graduates, and most of our respondents have been in the profession for one year, with a minimum of one month and a maximum of 10 years.*
- *The documents available to most pharmaceutical service providers are not complete enough to ensure the viability of the structure, and some find operating authorizations at the IPS, the DPS and religious denominations; whereas according to the regulations, all should come from the IPS.*
- *All pharmacies obtain their medicines and medical consumables from pharmaceutical wholesalers, with most not having a medicines and consumables management manual.*

Key words: Management, Drugs and medical consumables.

SUMMARY

With the rather worrying situation, on resistance to antibacterials, a study was carried out on pharmacies anarchically open to the public in the city of Bukavu and its surroundings; in order to identify the factors that contribute to the emergence of resistance from them...

Our proposal study was based on discribing and analysing the medicaments consuption and their gestion in the public drugstores within the Ibanda health zone to determin factors that influence negativelly treatment and servises in health care structure and suggest recomandations to erradicate that issue.

Sering the nationd policy that aims the efficient emprovement and the accessibility of sanitary structures many efforts had been conjugated but the results remain complex. The case of public drugstores Ibande health zone wich has health care services with health structures. Documentary analyse, observation and the chalking with drugstore assistants allowed and determined the the efficience and validity to discribe the medicaments process gestion and consumable medicaments in open in public of the Ibanda health zone, people implicated directly in medicaments gestion and their consurption within health structures, notably :

- ✓ *The majority of agents when work in the public drugstores are women assistants of drugstore in their twenties thirties and forties, but most of them are in their twenties and still strolents;*
- ✓ *All drugstores assistant are seemed to have less knowledge in medical sciences. specialy pharmacy; but what seves them is the experience that they have in that job about or around 10 years some of them;*
- ✓ *Some of drugstores assistant use document which are not only update but also which an no complet for the access of the structure and some find the functional allowences from ISP, DPS, religious confessions, ... while, reguarding the regulations all allowance should course from ISP;*
- ✓ *The drugestores in their totality are impoisoned in medicament use and consumption of médicamental products whithin sold institution (houses) though*

in balk or detail, assistant never despose a books of medicament gestion and consumption.

Key words: Management, Médicaments and consumable medicaments.

0.1. PROBLEMS

Antimicrobial chemotherapy in the 20th century represented a major step forward in infectious pathology. It revolutionized medical treatment, defeating diseases that contributed to great suffering, disability and death. Over time, more powerful antimicrobials have been produced and made available to the world for better treatment. However, many pathogens are increasingly developing resistance to antimicrobials, making effective treatment impossible. As this happens, epidemics may result in high morbidity and mortality. Antimicrobial resistance has largely contributed to the rise in morbidity and mortality from infectious and parasitic diseases over the past half-century. Antimicrobial resistance is therefore becoming a major public health issue.

Over the past half-century, the use of antimicrobials has made a major contribution to reducing morbidity and mortality from infectious and parasitic diseases. However, these results are increasingly compromised by the rapidly growing problem of resistance to these drugs. Infectious and parasitic diseases such as tuberculosis, sexually transmitted infections, acute respiratory infections, malaria, dysentery and HIV/AIDS have become increasingly difficult and costly to treat, resulting in a very heavy burden, particularly in developing countries where resources are very limited in the face of high infection rates. The rising costs of resistant infections are seriously undermining efforts to prevent, control and treat infectious and parasitic diseases worldwide, and jeopardizing the benefits of healthcare investments.

Drug resistance has emerged in all categories of pathogens: viruses, fungi, parasites and bacteria. Major pathogens that have become resistant to antimicrobials include :

- Bacteria that cause various infections, such as staphylococci, enterococci and E. Coli;
- Agents that cause respiratory infections, such as streptococcus pneumonia, tuberculosis and influenza;
- Food-borne pathogens such as Salmonella and Amylobacter;
- Sexually transmitted micro-organisms, such as Neisseria gonorrhoeae;
- Candida and other fungal infections ;
- Parasites, such as Plasmodium falciparum, the agent of malaria;
- Human Immunodeficiency Virus (HIV), the agent of AIDS. Factors

contributing to the acceleration of resistance include the ineffectiveness of chloroquine as a primary antimalarial, multidrug-resistant tuberculosis (MDR-TB) and extensively drug-resistant tuberculosis (XDR-TB), various antibiotic-resistant diarrheal diseases and acute respiratory infections, HIV/AIDS, and methicillin-resistant Staphylococcus aureus (MRSA). Numerous complex mechanisms of antifungal resistance have been observed, and antibacterial resistance has gradually gained ground, as in the case of :

1. Penicillin has lost much of its effectiveness against pneumonia, meningitis and gonococcal disease in many countries. In the USA, 80% of Staphylococcus aureus isolations are resistant to penicillin and 32% are resistant to penicillin;
2. Multi-resistant Salmonella infections are now a major public health problem in Asia;
3. Shigella resistance to ampicillin, tetracycline, cotrimoxazole and chloramphenicol is widespread in Africa, even though these drugs are still used for the first-line treatment of dysentery in many places. The introduction of nalidixic acid was followed by the emergence of resistance in Shigella ;
4. The emergence and spread of resistance in Salmonella dysenteriae type 1 to cotrimoxazole, ampicillin, tetracycline, chloramphenicol and, increasingly, nalidixic acid over the last twenty years means that these inexpensive and widely available antibacterials can no longer be used empirically;
5. Penicillin and erythromycin resistance is an emerging problem in community-acquired Streptococcus pneumoniae infections in Asia, Mexico, Argentina and Brazil, as well as in parts of Kenya and Uganda;
6. The spread of resistance in Neisseria gonorrhoeae has meant that penicillin and tetracycline have had to be replaced by more expensive second-line drugs, to which resistance has rapidly developed. In the Caribbean and South America, resistance to azithromycin was found to be 72% in many isolations from various locations, leading to recommendations to replace this drug with ceftriaxone, spectinomycin or quinolones. The high cost of other options, such as third-generation cephalosporins, makes their use prohibitive in many developing countries;
7. Antibacterial resistance to cholera is increasingly common in developing countries, with up to 90% of Vibrio cholerae isolations resistant to at least one antimicrobial.

Antibacterial resistance has a negative impact not only on therapeutic gain: antibacterial resistance increases morbidity and portability in patients with a wide range of diseases. The period of infectivity is prolonged, resulting in an increased risk of transmission of resistant micro-organisms. For example, a study of ultra-resistant tuberculosis carried out in South Africa in 2006 showed that 52 of the 53 cases identified died from the disease. These patients with resistant tuberculosis most certainly had the opportunity to transmit the disease to the other person.

Secondly, in economic terms: the cost of antimicrobial resistance to the individual and to society is enormous.

For example, treating multi-drug-resistant tuberculosis costs around 300 times more than treating non-drug-resistant tuberculosis. The cost of MRSA infection is triple that of penicillin-sensitive staphylococcal infections.

The use of second-line antimicrobials to treat resistant infections is not only more expensive, but can also lead to an increased incidence of unwanted resections.

Not only that, several mechanisms explain the occurrence of resistance, particularly in the case of malaria; chromosomal-type resistance, plansmid-type transmission, which are mutations causing a biochemical change that disrupts drug action (either by loss of receptor assertiveness, or by modification of drug transport and enzymatic changes altering metabolic activity), whereas in bacteria, mutations, generic transfer using transformation, conjugation, transduction or lysogenic conversion are generally reported.

However, it should be added that many factors contribute to resistance, including, among others, inappropriate prescribing by healthcare providers and inappropriate self-medication by patients; poor compliance with treatment is also an important factor contributing to drug resistance. In addition, limited access to healthcare, lack of regulation of antimicrobial availability, substandard or counterfeit products, poor storage conditions and inadequate infection control in healthcare facilities are all factors within the healthcare system that contribute to the emergence and spread of resistance.

The inventory of the pharmaceutical sector carried out in 2019 showed that of the 365 health facilities acting as GRHs that were surveyed, only 55, or 15%, had all the tracer drugs selected at the time of the survey. The availability of medicines is very limited in most health facilities in our country in general, and in South Kivu province in particular. Pharmacies open to the public are the alternative for drug availability. As such, their uncontrolled opening could compromise the quality of medicines dispensed to the population.

We conducted a study of anarchic pharmacies open to the public in the city of Bukavu, particularly in the Ibanda health zone, to identify the factors contributing to the emergence of antibacterial resistance.

Medicinal products are defined as any substance or composition represented as having curative or preventive properties with respect to human or animal diseases, as well as any substance or composition that can be used in humans or animals, or that can be administered in order to establish a medical diagnosis or to restore, correct or modify their physiological functions by exerting a pharmacological, immunological or metabolic action. People should expect to receive safe, quality health products, properly distributed at an affordable price. Health is a fundamental human right, and access to health care, which includes access to essential medicines, is an indispensable condition for the enjoyment of this right. Access to healthcare products to prevent infection or treat disease should not be a risky business (Frédéric D, P1, 2022).

Almost two billion people - a third of the world's population - do not have regular access to essential medicines. In some low-income countries in Africa and Asia, more than half the population is affected by this problem. Adopting better policies for purchasing, prescribing and ensuring the quality of medicines is a major source of savings in all countries. The use of generic medicines is very effective in this respect, and is specifically mentioned. According to the report, any policy that encourages the use of generic medicines can save around 60% of drug costs in many countries. Furthermore, the global pharmaceuticals market is neither transparent nor efficient. Prices paid for identical medicines vary considerably from one country to another. In many countries, patients pay far too much for their medicines, sometimes up to 60 times the reference price on the international market. Worldwide, around half of all medicines are prescribed, dispensed or sold inappropriately - one of the main causes of infant mortality in developing countries. Hospitals are another area where better management could generate considerable savings. The mismanagement of medicines, prescription errors and poor storage of medical consumables remains a great danger in the healthcare delivery sector, but is also fatal. (Tedros A ; p.14-15, 2010)

Despite ongoing support from UN member states and other international organizations over several decades, the lack of availability and high cost of essential medicines for the treatment of communicable diseases has been highlighted, and the WHO Global Plan of Action for the Control of Non-Communicable Diseases 2013-2020 sets a target of 80% availability and affordability of essential medicines needed to treat major non-communicable diseases in public and private facilities. Effective prevention, treatment and care require access not only to affordable quality medicines, but also to vaccines, diagnostic blood products and quality-assured devices. The global strategy adopted by the WHO to improve access to essential medicines is based on the following principles: evidence-based selection of a limited number of medicines, rational purchasing, affordable prices, efficient distribution systems and rational use of medicines. All these elements promote better medicine management, and their effective implementation will increase access to medicines, facilitate progress towards universal health coverage and the health-related Millennium Development Goals, and guarantee the effectiveness of treatment and care. (Zambara S. & all, p.3, 2014).

The pharmacy network is highly developed in the United States, with most supermarkets (Supeway, Target, Hyve, Walmmant) featuring pharmacy departments integrated with the others. Alongside these pharmacies, there are small independent pharmacies (officine pharmaceutique), much like in France: they are sometimes found in large cities, but sometimes also in small villages. They are quite rare... There are also very few so-called integrative pharmacies. The best-known chain is Pharmaca (present in the western states). The shelves of these chains are stocked with self-service drugs in apparent abundance, but the choice of medicines is relatively small. The shelves seem full, but it's often the same over-the-counter drugs that are reasonable, just as the prices of prescription drugs are exorbitant. Example: $160 for a cream that costs around €5 in France). But the price you have to pay depends heavily on your insurance coverage. Despite the Obamacare health insurance reform, social protection has not evolved for those already affiliated to a private health insurance scheme (Isabelle G. ; p.12, 2023).

In Europe, over 50% of medicines used to treat cancers, infections and nervous system disorders account for more than half of those in short supply. Between 2000 and 2018, shortages in the EU increased by a factor of 20 and, according to a Commission communication, shortages of essential medicines are on the increase. The health crisis caused by COVID-19 has highlighted a major problem: shortages of medicines and medical equipment that put patients' lives at risk and healthcare systems under pressure. In April 2020, the Alliance of European Teaching Hospitals predicted that the growing demand for anesthetics, antibiotics, muscle relaxants and off-label drugs in intensive care units to treat Covid-19 could lead to stock-outs. Declining production, logistical worries, export bans and stockpiling also increase the risk of bottlenecks forming. The European Parliament has passed a resolution urging the European Union to become more autonomous in the healthcare field, by securing supplies, boosting local drug production and coordinating EU health strategies more effectively. The reasons for the shortage are complex: manufacturing problems, industrial quotas, parallel sales markets, unexpected increases in demand and national pricing. The European Union is increasingly dependent on third countries (mainly India and China) for the production of active pharmaceutical ingredients, chemical materials and medicines. This has led to a shortage of medicines and medical consumables, which must be made available to the European community in the quality and quantity needed to guarantee good health. However, with this shortage of medicines, the proper management of pharmaceutical products remains a top priority for European countries to ensure adequate health preservation. (Aidas S., p.2-3, 2023).

In the Western world, the unavailability of essential medicines remains a cause for concern. Legislative, regulatory and professional measures have been taken to ensure the proper management and supply of medicines and medical consumables, but the effective implementation of shortage management plans for medicines of major therapeutic interest at the start of 2017 has not resolved the situation, and we are seeing a deterioration rather than an improvement in the availability of medicines at both French and European level. We're not talking here about new products whose non-availability is associated, more often than not, with economic problems of market access during the first years of their commercialization, but rather old products whose therapeutic use is well established and considered to be of major relevance. The causes of these supply disruptions are manifold, and require the coordination of many players to resolve. Drug supply disruptions are a genuine public health concern. Health professionals in all countries have observed a steady rise in the number of supply disruptions. This phenomenon, which affects both dispensing pharmacies and hospitals, concerns both new and old drugs, as well as generics. The problem is getting worse: in 2021, the ANSM received 2,160 reports of stock-outs and risks of stock-outs, compared with 405 in 2016, 1,504 in 2019 (and after 2,500 in 2020, at the height of the pandemic). At the end of December, China requisitioned the production of certain pharmaceutical companies, at a time when millions of Chinese are struggling to obtain basic medicines to treat themselves in the face of an unprecedented wave of Covid-19. (Marie-Christine K. & all., p.4, 2018).

In some developing countries, over 40% of health budgets are spent on pharmaceuticals, yet large sections of the population have no access to the essential medicines needed to prevent or treat prevailing diseases. The scarce resources available are frequently used to buy ineffective or even dangerous drugs, or drugs that may be of great benefit but have a significant impact on the economy. This is why all decisions concerning the selection of drugs, insofar as they enable more rational therapy, are of considerable importance. The development of an essential drug list and a national therapeutic formulary for public health programs is the best way to ensure that the nations of efficacy, safety and economy are taken into account by prescribers. The provision of essential medicines is one of the eight components of primary health care. (Albert T., p.11, 2004)

Access to quality medicines still faces many challenges on the African continent. Distribution chains are often fragmented, with multiple intermediaries or parallel channels that often fuel counterfeiting, a real public health issue. Almost 60% of medicines purchased in the Gulf of Guinea are classified as "SF" (substandard, falsified) by the WHO. And the problem is not confined to Africa, since 10% of all medicines in circulation worldwide could be SF. As for local production, it is still struggling to make a place for itself in an African pharmaceutical market 70% supplied by foreign imports and marked by difficulties of access to raw materials, particularly active ingredients, and constraints of customs clearance operations, unpredictable delivery times, etc.). South of the Sahara, with the exception of South Africa and Tanzania, it is difficult if not impossible to find active ingredient production units. Access to financing, the establishment of permanent industrial facilities, the lack of regulatory harmonization between countries and the availability of highly qualified personnel are further obstacles to the development of private players in the pharmaceutical industry on the continent. With 13% of the world's population but only 3% of global pharmaceutical production, and a majority of counterfeit medicines, the African continent faces a major public health challenge: access to affordable, quality medicines. A battle in which the private sector has a decisive role to play. The needs are as great as the sector's growth potential. Yet the African continent still lags far behind the world drug market. Pharmaceutical dispensaries play a major role in the supply of medicines and the provision of services to patients, as they do in the private sector (Marie-Paule K., p.2-7, 2018).

In sub-Saharan Africa there is a permanent gap between the demand and supply of medicines, according to a report by the United Nations Office on Drugs and Crime. The high prevalence of infectious diseases, including malaria, combined with the lack of availability of medicines, financial capacity of populations and access to healthcare, creates an environment in which the demand for medical products and services is not fully met by formal channels. This gap between demand and supply of regulated pharmaceutical products leaves room for trafficking, encourages the involvement of organized criminal groups and fuels the permanent threat to the security of the country's populations. As proof, between January 2017 and December 2021, at least 605 tonnes of different medical products were seized in West Africa during international operations, notes the United Nations Organization against Drugs and Crime, which points out that despite the lack of reliable information on the volumes of medicines involved, various studies estimate that between 19 and 50% of pharmaceutical products on the market in Sahel countries are falsified and of inferior quality. According to a report by the United Nations Office on Drugs and Crime, 270,000 people die every year in sub-Saharan Africa as a result of consuming falsified and substandard anti-malarial drugs. In addition, the deaths of 169271 children in the region are attributed to the use of counterfeit antibiotics to treat severe pneumonia in young patients. The figures are appalling, and highlight the terrible consequences of illicit trafficking and counterfeiting of medicines and medical equipment. (Zaina J., p.1-5, 2023).

In DR Congo, as in almost all developing countries, despite the efforts made to supply medicines and medical consumables over the last 30 years, the management of medicines and medical consumables in health facilities by those in charge of them is a problem for the entire minimum and complementary package. The rate of access to healthcare varies between 40% and 50%, according to the WHO's Demographic and Health Survey. Clearly, over 30 million Congolese do not have access to quality healthcare. Trend data from certain health zones show that rational management of medicines and medical consumables can increase significantly when the price of medicines drops (and their quality and quantity increases), thanks to the implementation of external aid programs. Despite multiple efforts by the DRC's Ministry of Health, the pharmacy sector remains constrained by various problems relating to medicines and medical consumables. In Ituri Province, the international medical organization Médecins Sans Frontières (MSF) reported in an article that over 1,000 people had been poisoned by falsified or mislabeled medicines. Ineffective drug regulation mechanisms, combined with inadequate penalties, corruption and porous borders, make poor communities easy prey for those who sell toxic, poor-quality medicines. These drugs call into question all the progress made in pharmacology and public health. The multiplication of serious cases by falsified medicines must make global or Public Health actors react and encourage them to ensure that patients in particular the most vulnerable are prescribed appropriate and good quality medicines and that they are able to obtain them (Dr Peyrand, P_2, 2017).

The socio-economic crisis that the country (DRC) has been going through for more than a decade means that a large part of the population has no access to essential medicines and medical consumables. In Kinshasa, the proliferation of pharmaceutical establishments granting medicines of inferior quality, at low prices and putting them in competition with CDR in general and in particular, this inaccessibility results from the high prices of medicines due to the level of taxes, logistical costs and the non-subsidization of medicines. In North Kivu, poor governance of the pharmaceutical system is one of the factors contributing to disparities in access to medicines, and in the public supply of essential, quality medicines. Not only does the Congolese government bear responsibility for the challenges facing the pharmaceutical sector, but also a range of individuals present at all levels play major roles in this sector. In the Democratic Republic of the Congo, as in other countries in sub-Saharan Africa, the use of healthcare services is still low and far from praiseworthy, according to the WHO, yet the use of basic healthcare services is one of the factors promoting better health for populations, along with the effectiveness of local structures such as health facilities and pharmacies. The population of the eastern part of the Democratic Republic of Congo lives in precarious health conditions. The worrying security situation, poverty and geographical and cultural particularities compromise the health care of many inhabitants. South Kivu province has the highest mortality rates in the country, particularly among mothers and children. In addition, malaria, acute respiratory infections, parasitic diseases and regular epidemics are all health problems for which the population would benefit from access to effective, high-quality medicines, taking into account socio-economic capacities. (Manya KK, P. 2 -5, 2023)

In South Kivu, a large number of pharmacies operate in an unprecedented environment. This way of working has led to the circulation of medicines and medical consumables with modified manufacturing dates on the province's black markets, which presents a danger for the local population. There's a pharmacy on every street corner in Bukavu, most of them run by non-experts. For many owners, all that's needed to get their pharmacy up and running is a capital sum, an operating license and a procès-verbal or authorization to open. It doesn't matter where these documents come from, or under what conditions pharmaceutical and medical products are sold and managed. (Fidèle M., p.3-6, 2014).

In the commune of Ibanda, pharmacies are hiding a lot of food and drink, and regulatory measures are vital to protect this sector and the population, who are being plundered by unsuitable and poorly preserved medicines. According to the South Kivu provincial pharmacy inspectorate, a pharmacist should be a member of the Order of Pharmacists and be qualified after official training recognized by the Congolese state. Despite the many efforts made by other managers to improve the management of medicines and medical consumables, there are still many negative factors. This raises the question:

- ✓ Do pharmaceutical dispensaries have the operating document for dispensing health care services?
- ✓ What profile does the pharmaceutical dispensary agent have to manage medicines and medical consumables properly?
- ✓ What is the source of supply of medicines and medical consumables for pharmacies?

0.2. HYPOTHESIS

- ✓ Pharmaceutical dispensaries are said to have false or non-existent operating documents for dispensing health care services;
- ✓ Pharmaceutical dispensary agents have profiles that are inconsistent or inappropriate for the pharmacy to ensure the proper management of medicines and medical consumables within the structure;
- ✓ The source of supply for drugs and medical consumables would be pharmaceutical wholesalers.

0.3. OBJECTIVE

0.3.1. General objective

In general, this work aims to contribute to the adequate and effective improvement of the management system for medicines and medical consumables in pharmaceutical dispensaries, and to initiate possible solutions for the rational management of medical materials and equipment in the Ibanda health zone.

0.3.2. Specific objective

- ✓ Analyze the operating document used by pharmacies to dispense healthcare services;
- ✓ Identify the profiles available to pharmacy agents;
- ✓ Evaluate the sources of supply of medicines and medical consumables for pharmacies.

0.4. CHOICE AND INTEREST OF SUBJECT

We have therefore chosen to carry out this study on the management of medicines and medical consumables within pharmaceutical dispensaries, in order to provide managers with up-to-date basic data, enabling them to initiate policies that offer the effectiveness of ensuring adequate, effective and sustainable management of medicines and medical consumables by the managers of these structures, in the interests of the well-being and good service guarantees offered in the community.

The data generated by the results of this study will open up new avenues of research for others who want to follow in our footsteps.

0.5. SUBJECT DELIMITATION

Spatially, our work focuses on the management of medicines and medical consumables in pharmaceutical dispensaries in the Ibanda health zone.

In terms of timing, this study covers the period from April 2023 to October 2023.

0.6. METHODOLOGICAL APPROACH

We carried out a descriptive, exploratory and retrospective study with a mixed approach, which enabled us to describe our study site; the systematic method, which enabled us to study the supply system for essential medicines in pharmaceutical dispensaries; the documentary analysis, which was important for enriching the present work by consulting the various documents relating to our research theme, i.e. books, course notes, etc.; direct observation, which enabled us to get a feel for the reality in the field; and the free interview, which enabled us to talk to the people in charge of the management or responsibility of the pharmaceutical dispensary, in order to obtain information about the situation in the field, direct observation, which enabled us to get a first-hand feel of the reality in the field; and free interviews, which enabled us to talk to those in charge of managing or responsible for the pharmaceutical dispensary, to obtain additional information on our subject.

0.7. LABOR SUBDIVISION

Apart from the introduction, the conclusion and the recommendations and suggestions, this work is subdivided into two parts: the theoretical part which focuses on :

- Chapter 1: Review of the literature on the management of medicines and medical consumables ;
- Chapter two: Methodology and materials

And the empirical section devoted to :

- Chapter three: Data collection and experimental phases ;
- Chapter four: Results and discussion.

Chapter 1: REVIEW OF THE LITERATURE ON DRUG AND MEDICAL CONSUMABLES MANAGEMENT

I.1. REVIEW OF THEORETICAL LITERATURE

I.1.1. Defining key concepts

a) **Pharmaceutical dispensary:** the place where pharmacists sell, store and prepare medicines. We go there after visiting the doctor (or a healthcare professional) with a prescription, or to buy self-service medicines and healthcare products. (module tout savoir sur l'officine de pharmacie, (La rousse, 2019)

b) **A medicine:** is any substance or composition presented as having curative or preventive properties with regard to human or animal diseases. By extension, a drug includes any substance or composition that can be used in or administered to humans or animals, with a view to establishing a medical diagnosis or to restoring, correcting or modifying their physiological functions by exerting a pharmacological, immunological or metabolic action (Drug Management Training Module, min santé 4).

c) **Essential drugs:** these are drugs that are essential for the health of the majority of the population. An indicative list, periodically updated, is drawn up by the WHO according to the local needs of developing countries. Essential medicines, as defined by the WHO, are those that meet the health needs of the majority of the population. (Article on WHO essential medicines)

d) **Generic drug:** a copy of an original drug whose production and marketing have been made possible by the expiry of the patent covering the drug. A generic drug is therefore an original or "originator" drug whose patent has expired after a 20-year monopoly, and which can now be manufactured by a company other than the one that invented it. In cases of emergency (e.g. a major fatal epidemic), "compulsory licenses", i.e. premature exceptions to the patent rule, are theoretically provided for. (Dr. Erold Joseph, 2023).

e) **Expired drugs:** these are drugs that have passed the expiration date indicated on the packaging. The expiration date of a pharmaceutical product depends on data from a sample library; this collection of samples indicates the date at which the degradation of active ingredients is too great for the product to remain effective, and the drug may also prove dangerous: for example, aspirin turns into two acids when it is expired, both of which can burn the oesophagus. The ageing of products is sometimes accelerated by the conditions in which they are preserved, particularly temperature, as some are more fragile than others. Unused medicines can be returned to your pharmacist, who will pass them on to Cyclamed, the organization responsible for destroying them. (Dr. Brigitte Blong, 2021).

f) **Medical equipment:** is defined as goods intended to remain permanently in the same form made possible in real time in quantity and quality intended for all hospital departments to all those who need them. Because of their lifespan, medical equipment is the type of material that lasts a long time and needs to be maintained and renewed. Their storage requires special attention from the depot or pharmacy to avoid their invalidity; the management of medical equipment is no different from that of medicines in a pharmacy (ECZ PHC management training module p.6).

g) **Pharmacy:** science applied to the design, preparation and distribution of medicines. In a local hospital, where drugs are stored and prepared for patients undergoing treatment. (Larousse). Pharmacy is the science concerned with the design, mode of action, preparation and dispensing of medicines. Dispensing takes into account possible drug interactions between chemical molecules, as well as interactions with edible products. It also enables us to check doses and/or any contraindications. It is a branch of biology, chemistry and medicine (Wikipedia).

h) **Medical devices management:** this covers all medical devices requiring calibration, preventive and corrective maintenance, user training and decommissioning-activities which are the responsibility of ordinary biomedical engineers. Medical equipment is used for the specific purpose of diagnosing and treating disease or injury, or rehabilitating patients, and may be used alone or in conjunction with auxiliary or consumable equipment, or other devices. Medical equipment does not include implantable, injectable or disposable medical devices. Medical equipment is also referred to in this document as "medical equipment", "healthcare equipment" or "material". (Module on Introduction to Medical Equipment Management WHO Technical Series on Medical Devices, p.4)

i) **Management:** comes from the verb to manage, which means to administer as manager. Gestion is therefore the action of managing, organizing something, directing; the period during which someone manages a business. (Larousse). Management pioneer Henry Fayol (1841-1925) explained the principles of global business management in his book "administrer, c'est pouvoir, organiser, commander, coordonner et contrôler". This was to ensure economical production, while eliminating waste and optimizing resources. According to Yves DUPUY, management, from the point of view of organizational practices, is the set of decision-making activities that take place in a company or, more generally, in an organization (administration, association, group, etc.). Managing therefore consists in choosing certain actions on the basis of varied information. Roumens, in turn, considers management to comprise three main actions: forecasting (budgeting), organization (data entry) and control (verification of forecasts). According to Charles Edouard, Séverine Godarol, le Petit Contrôle de gestion 2015, 6ème edition, Dunod, 2015. Managing a business or community organization means developing and implementing the tools that enable information to be shared, strategies to be discussed and decisions to be made transparently. Management enables the company's resources to be prioritized with a view to achieving predetermined objectives (sales, market share, etc.) within the framework of a given policy.

j) **To manage** is to use the resources at your disposal rationally or irrationally. It means managing and administering a stock of goods, information, computer data, a company, etc. (Larousse).

I.1.2. General information on the management of medicines and medical devices

Quality medicines and medical equipment save human lives and improve health, but only if they are available, affordable and properly used to meet the therapeutic needs of the majority of the population.

Despite this quantification of medicines, pharmacy owners or managers bring in medicines without taking into account the needs of the population, which is why many pharmaceutical products expire.

The tools for managing medicines and medical equipment in pharmaceutical dispensaries are available for some but not properly used, and others are non-existent or poorly maintained for the few who have them. The main causes are: stock sheets for medicines and equipment, inventory sheets, medicine use and revenue registers, supply registers, order donations and receiving reports:

- ✓ Absence of a manual of procedures for the management of medicines and medical materials ;
- ✓ Staff untrained in the management of medicines and medical equipment, as well as in pharmaceutical matters.

The stability and balance required for the successful delivery of healthcare services linked to the operationalization and distribution of medicines and medical devices as a whole depends on the rational and efficient management of supplies from stock and from manufacturer to user.

Effective stock management is necessary to avoid wastage and ensure continuity of supply. Stock procurement policy should be based on a detailed review of stock rotation records.

The main causes of ill-health in developing countries were demographic factors, malnutrition, sanitary conditions and housing, noted the World Bank in a document. Although the primacy of these factors is undeniable, and the reception they provoke and aggravate are directly more responsible for mortality, it is not necessary to wait for the improvement of these social conditions to prevent and treat these diseases which, in the majority of cases, can be cured or controlled thanks to the use of the necessary pharmaceutical products and equipment by qualified personnel.

I.1.3. Drug supply

In DR Congo, the Ministry of Health, with the support of its partners, set up the National Essential Drug Supply System (SNAM) in May 2002 to implement the National Pharmaceutical Policy. The SNAM's strategic orientation is to centralize drug procurement through two central purchasing coordination offices (in Kinshasa and Goma), and to decentralize distribution through regional drug distribution centers (CDR).

To promote and develop this system, the Ministry of Health created the National Essential Drug Supply Program (PNAM) in July 2002. Since 2002, the system has evolved, gradually meeting the challenge of geographic and financial accessibility of medicines at all levels of the health pyramid. However, with the increase in funds available for the treatment of priority diseases such as HIV/AIDS, malaria and tuberculosis, new players have emerged and are involved in the supply of medicines in DR Congo, sometimes with their own supply systems.

It is in this context, and in order to ensure a coordinated, coherent and efficient supply, that the Ministry of Public Health, in particular the Directorate of Pharmacy and Medicines (DPM) and the National Medicines Supply Program (PNAM), has requested WHO's support in mapping the supply and distribution of essential medicines and other health products in DR Congo.

The specific objectives of this mapping are :

- ✓ Identify and comprehensively analyze existing sources and systems offinancing, supply and distribution for essential medicines, including antiretrovirals, antimalarials, tuberculosis drugs, drugs for opportunistic infections, contraceptives, vaccines, condoms, laboratory reagents, medical devices, laboratory products and materials;
- ✓ Identify for each stage of the supply cycle (selection, quantification, purchasing, storage/stock management, distribution/dispensing, quality assurance system, financing, information management, monitoring/evaluation) and for each category of products studied:
    - Players/structures involved ;
    - Policies, strategies and tools used.

In South Kivu, logistics is the science of acquiring, storing and transporting medicines, medical consumables and small equipment. This involves the acquisition of products from CDR depots, for example, and the distribution of large quantities of medicines, medical consumables and small equipment at a given time, to a large number of health centers and medical-health services in different locations, as well as pharmaceutical dispensaries. This involves the actions and resources needed to acquire products, to deliver them to the place where they are needed, and to ensure that the right quality and quantity of product is delivered to the right place at the right time.

The activities involved in the process depend on each other, they are part of a system, a weakness in one part weakens the whole system. It's useful to think of our supply system in terms of four functions, four sets of activities. The logical supply cycle comprises :

- ✓ Selection ;
- ✓ Acquisition ;
- ✓ Distribution and ;
- ✓ Use.

Quality management runs through all four games. Diagram of Cycle 1

Selection-Acquisition-Distribution-Use

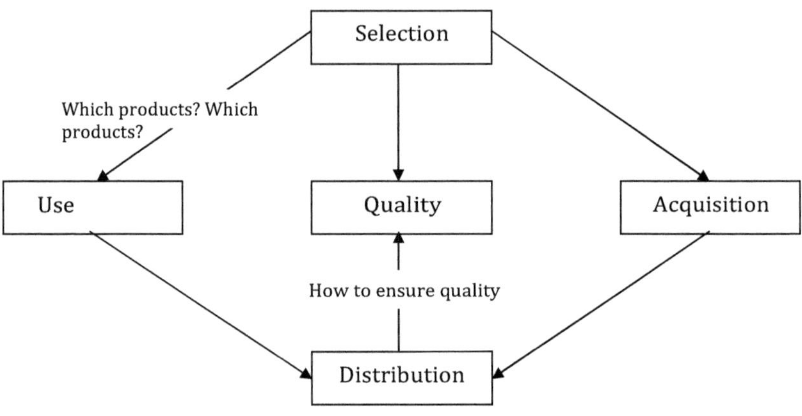

Figure 1: The supply cycle Packaging

- ✓ Prescription
- ✓ Dispensation
- ✓ Consumption control
- ✓ Which supplier?
- ✓ How to buy?
- ✓ How financial?
- ✓ Buying or manufacturing?
- ✓ Putting/keeping in stock
- ✓ Inventory management
- ✓ Replenishment
- ✓ Shipping

a) Selection: this involves determining which drugs should be available, and in what quantities.

Selection problems

- ✓ Selection of a wide variety of products
- ✓ Selection of unsuitable products
- ✓ Selecting expensive products in a low-income community
- ✓ Inappropriate quantity selection.

b) **Procurement:** this is the process of acquiring medicines, small equipment and medical consumables. It involves planning, deciding and implementing the method for obtaining the right quality and quantity of medicines. At this stage, you should be aware that :

- ✓ Which supplier to buy from?
- ✓ What price to buy?
- ✓ How to buy (cash or credit, etc.)
- ✓ Make or buy?
- ✓ How to finance (with what resources?)

Problems of acquisition

- ✓ Purchase of inappropriate quantities ;
- ✓ Unfavorable contract clauses (leonine contract)
- ✓ Inadequate financing (budget shortfalls, especially in foreign currency)
- ✓ Rare suppliers
- ✓ The poor performance of attention to quality assurance.

c) Distribution: at this stage, medicines must be received, stored, stocked and transported. Procurement, shipping and receiving take place at this stage.

The problems of distribution are :

- ✓ Poorly organized transport system
- ✓ Poor inventory management
- ✓ Poor storage conditions
- ✓ Poor information management

d) Utilization: includes aspects such as product packaging and labeling, as well as prescribing, dispensing, administration and consumption.

The following problems are encountered during use:

- ✓ Incorrect packaging and labelling
- ✓ Poor patient compliance
- ✓ The excessive cost of medicines, making healthcare inaccessible
- ✓ Administering or dispensing males to patients
- ✓ Irrational prescription.

I.2. REVIEW OF EMPIRICAL LITERATURE

The literature we have obtained has shown that the management of medicines and medical devices in pharmaceutical dispensaries is a cycle which begins with the selection of products (medicines and devices) to be ordered or requisitioned; followed by the supply of these medicines or medical devices, then distribution and finally use for patients or anyone else in need. (Drug and equipment management module, p.2). The various studies already carried out have produced the following results:

1. In Algeria, at the Université Mouloud Mammeri de Tizi-Ouzou, a study carried out in 2016-2017 on "drug management in hospitals: between perceived needs and availability - case study of the Chu de Tizi-Ouzou", prepared by : Boudjemai Thafsut showed that as part of contributing to improving the availability of drugs at Chu de Tizi-Ouzou that he had the description and analysis of the circuit of drugs at the hospital pharmacy. The mismatch between orders and the real needs of departments, the absence of an information system to ensure product traceability, the distribution of stocks between teams, and the lack of training in drug management are all points to be improved to ensure better drug availability and better meet patients' needs. In terms of results, the study revealed that the coverage of needs in terms of medicines differs from one product to another, which is due to several reasons (non-prescription, forecasting of departmental needs, nursing staff habitual, poor organization at departmental level and orders not reflecting real needs). To improve the availability of medicines in hospitals, we need to take action on the various stages of the drug supply chain, which are interdependent, not forgetting the people involved.
2. In Morocco in the national school of public health in health administration and public health the study carried out from 2012-2014 on the "analysis of the management of drugs and medical devices at the level of hospital pharmacy case of the Chp of Fes (Alghassani). Work prepared by M. Benjilali. Has shown that as part of the wide-ranging national policy to improve the availability of

medicines, several efforts are being made. In the same vein, this study sets out to describe and analyze the pharmaceutical product management circuit at Alghassani Hospital, in order to determine the factors that negatively influence their availability and propose recommendations. The results show that Alghassani Hospital devotes 53% of its operating budget to the purchase of pharmaceutical products and medical equipment. In the absence of data on consumption and traceability of products administered, quantification of needs is carried out at department level on an estimated basis and without any basis for calculation. In the absence of a computerized pharmaceutical product management application, average consumption and safety stock are not determined. Out of 331 products, 88 were out of stock (26.6%), and 69.3% of items were out of stock for long periods. 30 of the 53 out-of-stock medicines are life-saving.

3. In Kinshasa, at the Institut Supérieur des Techniques Médicales, the study of management and supply of essential medicines carried out in 2019, work done by kwete Minga. Concerns raised by the study centered on the following hypotheses: with regard to the supply of essential medicines, the weak points recorded show that the supply of essential medicines to the Ndjili HGR is not done properly; then, the standards for the management of essential medicines at the Ndjili HGR are not respected, due to the fact that the hospital does not obtain supplies from the CDR or BCZS, but rather from private depots. Secondly, standards require that all staff working in the pharmacy must be involved, but this is not the case at HGR Ndjili. Finally, in addition to product storage and stock shortages, other problems have been noted in the management and supply of essential medicines at the Ndjili HGR, notably the selection of supplies, inadequate lighting, and so on.
4. According to Antoine Mouhilo, who has worked on the management of medicines and medical equipment, the results are as follows: 39.85% of the operating budget is allocated to the purchase of pharmaceutical products, which is lower than the national average (45%) in Morocco. The survey of a sample of 489 patients revealed that: of the 489 patients, drug coverage is 100% for 345 patients, or 70.55% of patients. For the remaining 144 patients, they had to buy at least one drug, as coverage was only partially assured for prescribed treatments. Of the 1278 drugs prescribed to the 489 patients admitted to the emergency department, availability was only 100% assured for 1095 drugs, or

85.68% of prescribed drugs. Of the 183 drugs unavailable in the emergency department, 31% are due to stock-outs, and 25% are due to out-of-nomenclature prescriptions.

5. In Belgium, at the University of Liège, a study was carried out between 2022 and 2023 on "Managing drug stocks in hospital pharmacies: an analysis of the difficulties encountered in general hospitals in Wallonia", by Alexandre BARA. The main findings of this study reveal the difficulty of managing stock shortages, the complexity of keeping stocks up to d a t e , a lack of staff in care units and pharmacies, and the laborious management of return flows. This research has enabled us to identify various avenues for improvement to solve these problems. In the short term, these ideas could be applied in every hospital, thus resolving some of the complexities associated with inventory management. However, in the longer term, we believe that the current change in the Belgian hospital landscape is a real lever for more comprehensive solutions. Sharing data between member establishments would provide better visibility of the hospital environment, which could improve the anticipation and management of stock-outs, for example.
6. According to Yohane Kabwende François, for his work in Kadutu, he has proved the supply of medicines to large parts of households;

- ✓ For the majority of the population (93%), buying is the main way of obtaining medicines, as is the case for those who have a family pharmacy;
- ✓ The majority of households behave well, i.e. they buy their medicines at the pharmacy (86.6%). The majority of the population buys medicines without prescriptions, as can be seen from the fact that the many studies carried out have focused on the availability of essential generic medicines, sometimes on their accessibility, or even on their use, and others on the evaluation of the logistics system, without looking into the analysis of the management of essential generic medicines (p.20).

Our study differs from others in that it focuses on "the management of medicines and medical consumables in pharmaceutical dispensaries open to the public in the Ibanda health zone from May 2023 to October 2023", with the aim of improving the system for managing medicines and medical equipment in health facilities, in order to identify possible solutions for the rational and sustainable management of medical materials, medicines and equipment in DR Congo.

Method used: we adopted a descriptive, quantitative approach with analysis using appropriate statistical tools and a survey questionnaire.

I.3. CONCEPTUAL AND THEORETICAL FRAMEWORK

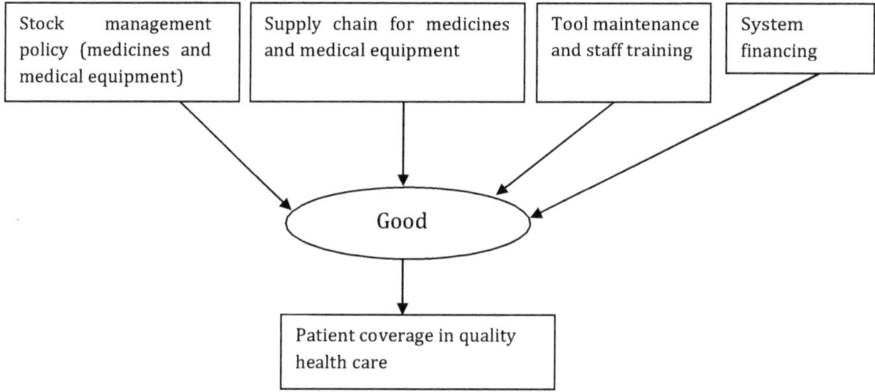

Chapter two: METHODOLOGY

II.1. Presentation of the study site

Our study was conducted in the Ibanda health zone in the commune of Ibanda, in the city of Bukavu, in the province of Sud-Kivu, in the Democratic Republic of Congo.

The Ibanda health zone is entirely within the urban area of the city of Bukavu.

A. Geographical location

The Ibanda health zone is one of thirty-four health zones in South Kivu province. It resulted from the 2003 division of the former Bukavu urban health zone into 3 health zones: Bagira, Ibanda and Kadutu. It is identified by the code 06010202. It covers an area of 18km^2 . It is bounded by :

- ✓ To the north by Lake Kivu ;
- ✓ To the north-west via the Kahuwa river and the ver "deux poteaux" industrial road, passing through Independence Square, the border with the Kadutu health zone;
- ✓ To the south, the Mulonge River separates it from the Nyatende health zone;
- ✓ To the east by the Ruzizi river, border with Rwanda ;
- ✓ To the west, by the Mbongwe mountain range and the overlap with the Bagira commune (Chai district).

It is mountainous, with clay soil and grassy vegetation, and a tropical climate. It has two seasons: the rainy season (September to April) and the dry season (May to August). It lies at an altitude of 1,200 to 1,800 meters and latitude 22°. The road is the access route and all its health areas are accessible.

B. Socio-economic situation

The Ibanda health zone covers an estimated population of 425,799, with a density of 23,656 inhabitants per square kilometer.

The population's main occupations, in descending order, are civil servants, petty traders and self-employed civil servants;

For family consumption, it depends on the availability of livestock products (meat, fish, milk), agricultural products (manioc, corn, beans, rice, vegetables, potatoes, fruit, etc.); and those derived from industrial processing and imports (soft and alcoholic drinks, juices, beer, sardines, mayonnaise, cookies, canned foods, etc.).

Repeated wars, especially in eastern DR Congo, have led to massive involuntary population movements from insecure areas (villages) to areas considered secure (towns). This has weakened the healthcare system, the security system, agricultural activities and the commercial system in South Kivu Province, without sparing the Ibanda health zone.

C. Cultural situation

The population of the Ibanda health zone is a symbiosis of tribes. The main ethnic groups are the Bashi, Lega, Bembes and Fulero. Swahili, Mashi and Kilega are the main local languages spoken.

The main religions are Catholic, Protestant, Muslim, Kimbanguist and Jehovah's Witness. Despite the health structures available to the population, they continue to turn to prayer rooms, herbalists and traditional practitioners in search of miracle solutions to their problems, even those requiring the advice of a health professional.

D. Health situation

The Ibanda health zone comprises twenty medical facilities, including two state health centers, eleven church health centers, one private health center, two state hospital centers, two church hospital centers, one accredited private hospital center and one general referral hospital.

I.2. Population

The population of the Ibanda health zone has grown from 21,2901 in 1985 to 515,834, distributed by health area as follows:

N°	Health area	Population
01	CECA 40 NGUBA	29877
02	CHAHI	36674
03	CIDASA	59176
04	NYAWERA	21557
05	GIHAMBA	27562
06	LABOTTE	15109

07	IRAMBO	17120
08	KABUYE	21910
09	MALKIA WA AMANI	25073
10	MAMAN MWILU	59137
11	MUHUNGU DIOCESAN	22478
12	MUHUNGU STATE	44201
13	CROIX-ROUGE	22683
14	PANZI	39164
15	MULUNGULUNGU	15571
16	VAVASORI	26669
17	NGUBA	31874
Total		**515 834**

Source: Zonal Central Office (ZCO) status 2023

Our study population consists o f a sample of all pharmacies in this section.

II.2. METHOD AND MATERIALS

II.2.1. Type of study

This is a descriptive, cross-sectional study.

II.2.2. Study material

To carry out our end-of-cycle work in health institution management, we used the following materials:

- ✓ A survey questionnaire addressed to managers directly involved in the management of medicines and medical devices within pharmaceutical pharmacies;
- ✓ IT tools: computer and printer for data entry and printing
- ✓ A diary and a pen to record any recommendations or elements relating to the management or operation of the structure.

II.2.3. Sampling method and technique

II.2.3.1. Sampling technique

This is both a non-probability sample of the opportunistic type, and a distribution cotat sampling technique.

II.2.3.2. Study population

a) Target population

Set of pharmacy agents on the management of the pharmaceutical dispensary.

b) Sample

According to expert opinion, we selected our sample on the basis of two criteria:

- ✓ Inclusion criteria: Our sample included all pharmacy staff directly involved in the management of medicines and medical devices through their daily tasks;
- ✓ Non-inclusion criteria: those not included in our sample are all people not directly involved in the day-to-day management of medicines and medical devices in pharmaceutical pharmacies.

c) Ethics

Our study protocol had been sent to the Ibanda BCZS and the required administrative authorizations had been obtained. Informed consent was obtained from all subjects who participated in our study. The motivations and objectives of the present study had been properly explained to them. They were reassured of the strict confidentiality of all data, and were informed about the dissemination of results after the survey.

II.2.4. Definition and operationalization of variables

A. Dependent variable

Management of medicines and medical consumables: this is a process that involves the selection, acquisition and distribution of materials (consumables) or medicines, with emphasis on quality and quantity, in order to avoid overstocking, stock-outs or product destruction.

B. Independent variable

1. Training in the management of medicines and medical equipment: this is an efficient process which ensures that medical products or consumables are available to patients (or those in need of them) throughout the pharmacy's service offering:

- ✓ Always have a minimum stock of medicines and medical consumables on hand to avoid stock-outs and over-stocking;

- ✓ Regular information on stock levels;
- ✓ Orderly arrangement and placement of items;
- ✓ Prepare orders based on physical stock;
- ✓ Avoid losses and out-of-date products;
- ✓ To prescribe medicines correctly, and to explain to patients when and how to take them;
- ✓ Prepare correct packaging when dispensing to the patient, to protect and facilitate proper administration of the drug (management manual and procedure 15p).

2. Manual of procedures for the management of medicines and medical devices: this procedural module is an essential working tool for establishing sound, transparent management and thus ensuring the sustainability of the healthcare chain. Finally, it constitutes a reference document for all operators (governmental institutions, NGOs, the UN, etc.) called upon to intervene in the field.
3. Management tool: a set of documents or software used on a day-to-day basis to manage, administer, direct and organize the company's day-to-day activities, with a view to deploying the company's resources to achieve pre-determined objectives, within the framework of a given policy (general chart of accounts).
4. Maximum stock: this is the level above which stock becomes excessive. In this case, we can speak of overstocking.
5. Month of supply: this is the regular time interval between two orders of essential generic medicines under normal conditions, i.e. in the absence of any threat of shortage.

   $$\text{MAD} = \frac{\textit{stock disponible}}{\textit{consommation moyenne mensuelle}}$$

6. Average monthly consumption (AMC): the average monthly consumption of a product is the number of units that the facility uses during a month; consumption may increase or decrease from month to month. Consequently, average monthly consumption (AMC) is the quantity that is calculated to be consumed during a month (Medication Management Manual p.16).

   $$\text{CMM} = \frac{\textit{consommation N mois}}{\textit{N mois}}$$

   $$\text{CMM corrected} = \frac{\textit{consommation de la période}}{\textit{la même période -jour de rupture de stock}}$$

7. Minimum or cover stock: this is the stock needed to meet customer requirements during the replenishment period.

   Minimum stock = DL x CMM + safety stock

8. Maximum stock: this is the maximum stock the pharmacy can hold at the beginning of the period. It must be evaluated taking into account product expiration dates, and is calculated using the formula :

   Max stock = CMM x 2

9. Safety stock: this is the reserve that ensures that products are always available in the event of a stock shortage. This stock is used to cover consumption between 2 orders (normally one month). It is also called reserve stock or buffer stock. It protects against possible stock-outs, if deliveries are late or if working stock is consumed faster than expected. It sets the threshold below which available stock must never fall.

   Safety stock $= \frac{stock d'alerte}{2}$

10. Alert stock: it is essential to have the supplies needed for the health service on hand at all times. Stock shortages (stock=0) always disrupt the smooth running of the department to a greater or lesser extent. To avoid stock-outs, the stock sheet includes an indicator: the alert stock, i.e. the quantity of supplies needed to reach the next delivery when the quantity available in stock reaches the alert stock quantity. At this point, you need to place an order, otherwise you run the risk of running out of stock

    Alert stock = CMM x 15

11. Out-of-stock: this is the absence of a molecule from the shelves of health facilities for a period of time. The drug must be usable, i.e. not expired. This absence is determined on the basis of the drug's stock record. 1,23
12. Available stock: this is the stock of products that can be used without danger to health.
13. Depreciation: this is the annual accounting recognition of the loss in value of a company's assets due to wear and tear, time or obsolescence. Depreciation spreads the cost of an asset over its useful life.
14. Provisions: this is a liability item. It represents an expense recorded in the current year, but for which the due date and/or amount are not yet known. Its inclusion in a company's balance sheet enables it to produce the most accurate accounting records possible. There are generally two types of provisions. Provisions for liabilities and charges arise from certain (for charges) or probable (for risks) obligations to third parties. They correspond to outflows of resources for which neither the amount nor the due date are yet fixed. Regulated provisions, on the other hand, are tax-driven and mainly concern provisions for price rises and investment provisions.

    Provision $= \frac{valeur\ d'acquisition\ x\ 20}{100}$

II.2.5. Data collection procedure

Four techniques were used to collect data: document review, observation, interviews and questionnaire. The questionnaire was first pre-tested:

- ✓ Observation using a grid: this was carried out in the pharmaceutical dispensary to check compliance with storage standards and the list of essential medicines displayed, as well as the organization and conservation of medicines and medical consumables.
- ✓ Semi-structured interviews: semi-structured interviews were used to identify and describe the drugs and medical consumables circuit. They were conducted on the basis of an individual interview guide with the managers of the pharmacies.
- ✓ The questionnaires: were distributed to staff in charge or managers of departments or involved in the management of medicines and medical consumables within pharmaceutical pharmacies.
- ✓ The pre-survey: enabled us to determine the management problems and select the pharmacies from which we gathered the necessary information.

In short, the study consisted of :

- ✓ Analysis of the management system for medicines and medical consumables in pharmaceutical dispensaries in the Ibanda health zone;
- ✓ The availability of medicines and medical consumables in pharmacies;
- ✓ Calculation and analysis of some important management data and indicators: corresponding drug requirements and the rate of depreciation of consumables;
- ✓ Description of the actual and current circuit of medicines and medical consumables in pharmaceutical pharmacies and the factors affecting their availability;
- ✓ Consultation of management tools: delivery notes, stock records, receiving reports, purchase orders and inventory, depreciation records;
- ✓ To ensure the availability and correct use of management tools.

II.2.6. Data processing and analysis

To analyze the data, we used the tools according to the component to be analyzed summarized in the table below:

Quantitative data analysis	Analysis of qualitative data
We used Word 2010 and Epi info to : Data entry ; Describe in percentage terms by Epi info, the calculation of CMM, MAD, DL, alert stock, etc. using predefined formulas.	Descriptive and comparative analysis The drug and medical consumables management process Transcription of semi-structured interviews ; Corpus coding and establishment of themes and sub-themes ; Vertical analysis by interview followed b y a cross-sectional analysis ; In-depth analysis and interpretation of themes; management of medicines and medical consumables: selection, reception, storage, stock management, distribution and storage. use.

Data triangulation has made it possible to obtain more reliable results, and has helped to improve stock management of medicines and medical consumables.

II.2.7. Subsequent results

On a practical level, the results obtained from this study can be used by public decision-makers, hospital managers and executives to overcome the challenges associated with the management of medicines and medical consumables.

These same results could be used as a reference in drawing up action plans to improve current processes. They present a detailed mapping of different processes relating to the management of medicines and medical consumables in pharmacies

II.2.8. Limits and difficulties encountered

This study focused on the analysis of the management of medicines and medical consumables and encountered difficulties such as :

- ✓ Search time reduced to a minimum;
- ✓ The doubts and sometimes carelessness of certain managers of the structures to provide us with all the information relating to the management of the medicines at our disposal;
- ✓ The lack of financial resources available to us to carry out this work. To overcome these difficulties, we capitalized on the means and time available to us for data collection, and were transparent with the respondents to avoid any doubts.

Chapter three: RESULTS

3.1. SOCIO-DEMOGRAPHIC CHARACTERISTICS

Table 1: Socio-demographic characteristics

Socio-demographic characteristics	Workforce (n=313)	%	Median (Min-Max)
Gender			
Female	162	51,8	
Male	151	48,2	
Age			
19 to 24 years old	57	18,2	27 years old (ages 19-53)
25 to 49 years old	254	81,2	
50 and over	2	0,6	
Marital status			
Divorced	1	0,3	
Widowed	4	1,3	
Married	146	46,6	
Single	162	51,8	
Study level			
Without	1	0,3	
Primary	3	1	
Secondary	67	21,4	
University	242	77,3	
Religion			
Others to be specified	5	1,6	
Jehovah's Witnesses	5	1,6	
Muslim woman	5	1,6	
Kimbanguist	9	2,9	
Protestant	144	46	
Catholic	145	46,3	
Other religion (n=5)			
Brahmin	4	80	
Neon apostolic	1	20	

This table shows that most of the respondents are women, and during the course of the survey we found that it is women who work more in pharmacies. The majority are aged between 25 and 49, and the median age is 27. Most of them have a university degree, and only one respondent said he had no formal education,even though he works as a pharmacist.

3.2. PROFILES OF PHARMACEUTICAL DISPENSARY AGENTS

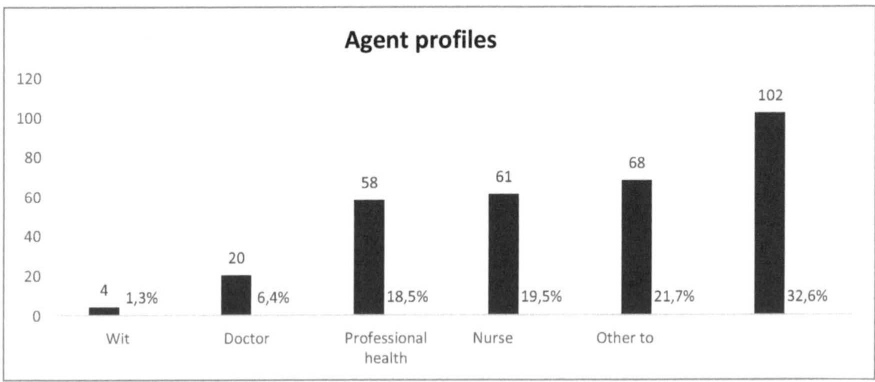

Figure 1: Pharmacy clerk profile

This figure shows that the majority of pharmacists have a good profile, as they have a background in the health sector, with a low proportion having studied pharmaceutical sciences.

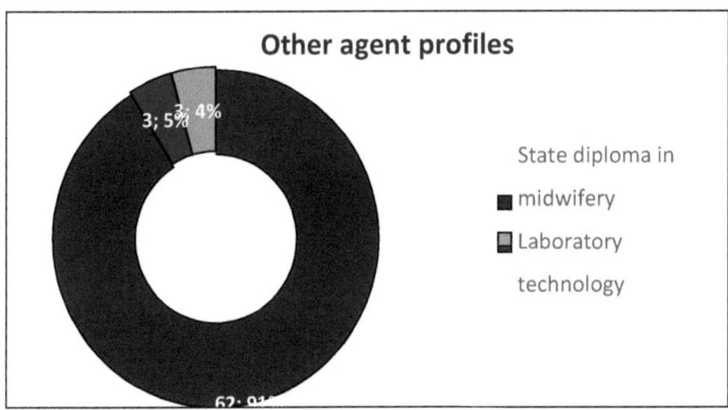

Figure 2: Other agent profiles at the pharmacy

Some pharmacists operate with a low profile and no knowledge or understanding of pharmacy. This just goes to show that the quality of service offered by these people leaves a lot to be desired.

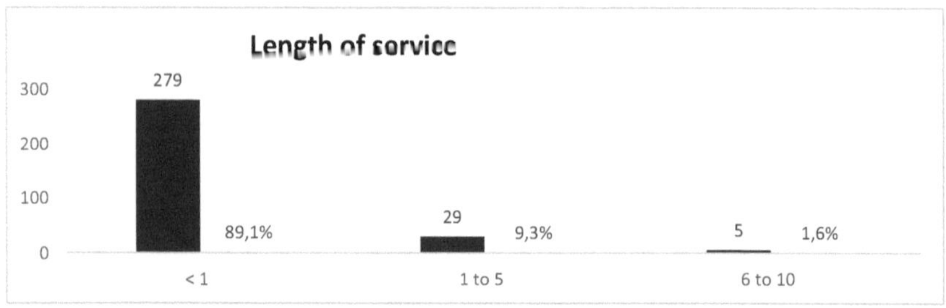

Most of our respondents have been pharmacists for less than a year, with a median of 7 months and a maximum of 10 years.

3.3. OPERATING DOCUMENT FOR SERVICE DELIVERY

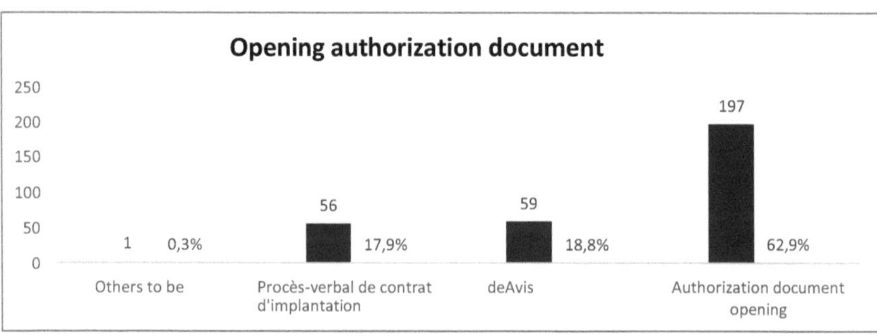

Figure 3: Operating documents for dispensing care

The document most pharmacists have at their disposal is the authorization to open, and it turns out that pharmacies don't have all the documents they need tbe viable.

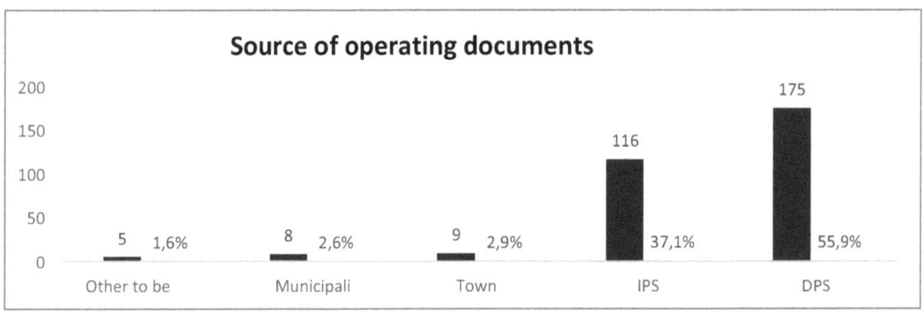

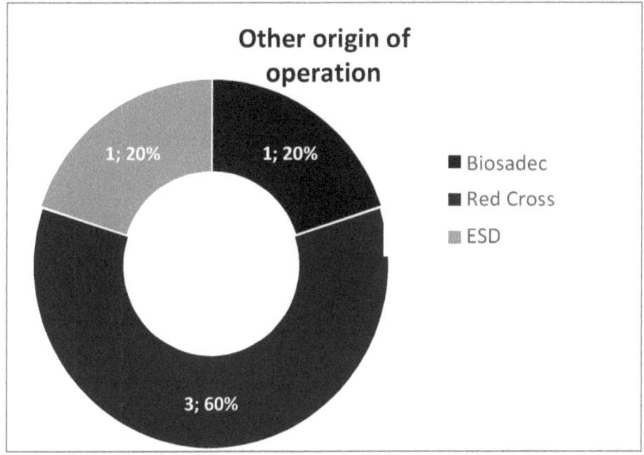

Figure 4: Origin of operating documents for service offering

Most pharmacies obtain their operating authorizations from the DPS and others from the IPS. Although a good proportion of people use the authorized services, just as many work in the informal sector, and this affects the quality of service provided by the latter.

3.4. SOURCES OF SUPPLY FOR DRUGS AND MEDICAL CONSUMABLES

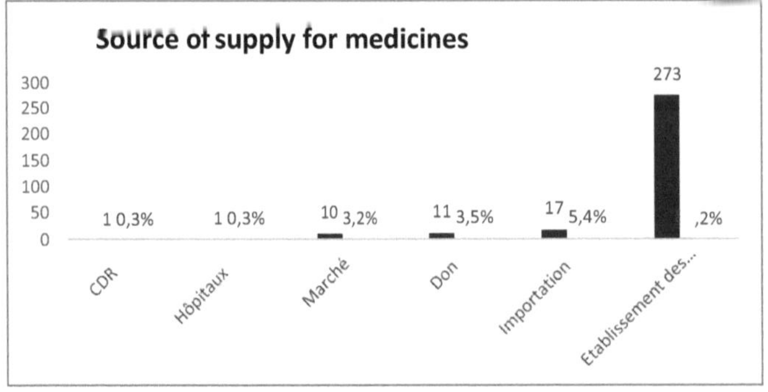

Figure 5: Source of supply for drugs and medical consumables

The source of supply for medicines and medical consumables is pharmaceutical wholesalers, according to most of the pharmacies surveyed.

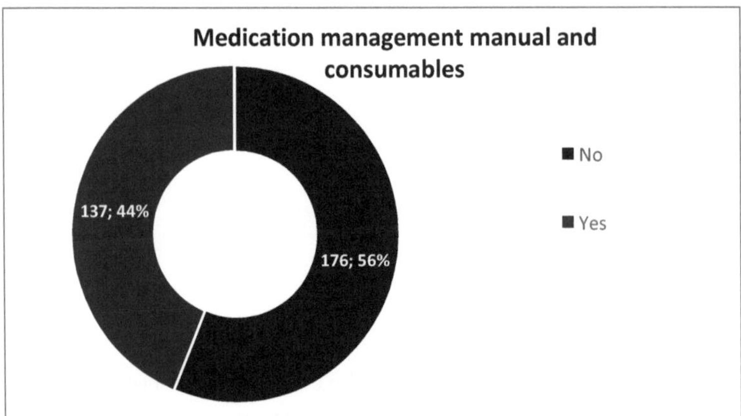

Figure 6: ***Drug and consumables management manual***

Most pharmacists do not have a drug and consumables management manual.

Chapter Four: DISCUSSION

The results of our study stand out from the others in that we analyze the management of medicines and medical consumables in pharmaceutical dispensaries open to the public in the Ibanda health zone, from which the following findings emerged. In our study of 313 service providers in pharmaceutical dispensaries, we found that :

- Our socio-demographic characteristics:

It emerges that women are more likely than men to be the providers in pharmacies open to the public in the Ibanda health zone, and this could be explained by the fact that men are more versatile in their activities in different professions than women, who remain more normal and sedentary.

The 25 to 49 age bracket remains in the majority in the pharmaceutical dispensaries open to the public in the Ibanda health zone, and the median age is 27. We understand that most are over the age of secondary school but at least university-educated, ready to move on to professional activities, while others have either the experience or the ability to do and launch themselves into the pharmaceutical service while still at university or having finished their studies.

University level education is the most abundant, making up a maximum majority of service providers in pharmaceutical dispensaries open to the public in the Ibanda health zone, followed by providers with secondary level education, and in lesser cases a pharmaceutical service provider with no level of education but who struggles in this profession.

It was found that the providers of pharmaceutical services in the Ibanda health zone are the most single, and most of them are still too young, but married people also represent a considerable proportion of the providers of services in pharmaceutical dispensaries open to the public. Catholic and Protestant Christians dominate, making up the maximum number of providers in pharmaceutical dispensaries open to the public in the Ibanda health zone, compared with other religions combined.

- Profile:

Most pharmaceutical service providers have a good profile, as they are trained in the medical and health fields, but there is a low proportion among them who have studied pharmaceutical science. However, some pharmaceutical service providers open to the public in the Ibanda health zone operate with a low profile and have no knowledge or understanding of pharmacy, which proves that the quality of service offered by these providers remains to be desired.

From the seniority or length of service of pharmaceutical dispensaries open to the public in the Ibanda health zone, we can see that most of our respondents have been in business for at least one year, with a median of 7 months, a minimum of one month and a maximum of ten years.

- Operating documents for dispensing pharmaceutical services:

The document most pharmacies open to the public in the Ibanda health zone have in their possession is the authorization to open, but not all pharmacies have all the documents they need to be fully viable. The majority of pharmacies open to the public obtain their operating authorizations from the provincial health division (DPS) and the fewest from the provincial health inspectorate, but there are also some that obtain their authorizations from other state institutions that do not cover health and under-coverage health institutions; although there is a good proportion of people who rely on skilled services, there are also just as many who work informally, and this affects the quality of service provided by providers in pharmacies open to the public.

- Source of supply of medicines and medical consumables;

Medicines and medical consumables for pharmacies open to the public in the Ibanda health zone are sourced from pharmaceutical wholesalers, commonly known as pharmaceutical depots, while a small number of pharmacies operating in the Ibanda health zone source their supplies from other locations. It is clear that most service providers do not have a drug and medical consumables management manual, yet its usefulness remains considerable given the appropriate arrangement, the layout according to the necessary standards of the pharmaceutical dispensary and the location of drugs and medical consumables for the layout of the pharmaceutical dispensary.

Thus, most service providers in pharmaceutical dispensaries open to the public in the Ibanda health zone deliver medicines and medical consumables by customer explanation during testing or consultation are those who direct a service provider to deliver a patient the right and precise pharmaceutical item while a patient may or may not well express or explain the effects he or she is experiencing. There is therefore a low rate of pharmaceutical service providers who deliver medicines and medical consumables by medical prescription or medical order; there is also a lower quantity of pharmaceutical service providers who deliver pharmaceutical items after test or consultation, and this is the case for providers in the capacity of nurse or doctor.

In view of the above, the management of medicines and medical consumables is not being carried out effectively and in accordance with standards in the Ibanda health zone, in pharmaceutical dispensaries open to the public.

A number of studies have analyzed the management of medicines and medical consumables, the causes being diverse. Problems in the management of medicines and medical consumables involve the training and information of the provider, the viability of the dispensary and the maintenance of support enabling the management and layout of medicines and medical consumables.

Boudjemai Thaysut from the University of Mouloud Nammeri in Tizi-Ouzou, Algeria, working on the management of medicines in hospitals in 2016-2017, compared to our study and results, showed that the lack of training in medicines management is one of the points to be improved to ensure better availability of medicines and better coverage of patients' needs.

The second is the work done by Kwete Mianga on the study of the management and supply of essential medicines carried out in 2019 at the Institut Supérieur de Techniques Médicales, which, similar to our results, showed that the supply of essential medicines at the HGR de Njili is not carried out properly, secondly, the standards for the management of essential drugs at the Njili HGR are not respected, due to the fact that the hospital does not obtain supplies from the CDR or BCZS, but rather from private depots.

The third case, similar to our result, comes from Yohane Kabwende's work in Kadutu, where he demonstrated that the majority of households buy medicines without a prescription, even though the majority of manages behave well, i.e. they buy medicines at the pharmacy (86.6%).

The fourth case is that of Bnejilali M at the national school of public health in health administration, the study carried out from 2012 - 2014 on the analysis of the management of drugs and medical devices at the level of hospital pharmacy case of (HP of FES alphasani), showed compared to our results that in the absence of data on consumption and traceability of products administered, the quantification of needs is done at the level of services in an estimated way and without basis for calculation. In the absence of a computerized pharmaceutical management application, average consumption and safety stock are not determined.

GENERAL CONCLUSION

With the aim of contributing to the improvement of the management of medicines and medical consumables in pharmaceutical officers open to the public in the Ibanda health zone, we have described and analyzed the management of medical products and consumables within pharmaceutical dispensaries open to the public to enable us to refute or confirm our hypotheses.

In view of the results, we can safely confirm that :

Pharmaceutical dispensaries do not have all the necessary accreditation documents to operate a pharmaceutical service, given the absence of all the documents required for the formal opening of a pharmaceutical dispensary (Figure 3). But there are also many people still working in the informal sector, and this affects the quality of service provided by the latter.

Our 2ème hypothesis is confirmed by the low number of people who have studied pharmaceutical sciences and yet are considered to be the ideal specialists and people to practice the art of pharmacy (Figure 1 and 2). Some pharmaceutical service providers perform this function with a low profile and no skills. This shows just how poor the quality of service offered by these providers really is.

The 3ème assumption that wholesalers are the source of supply for medicines and medical consumables is totally confirmed by the fact that all pharmacies source their supplies from wholesalers (Figure 5).

In terms of the results of the survey carried out among a sample of 313 pharmaceutical service providers in the Ibanda health zone, the management of medicines and medical consumables is not well assured. One of the objectives of the 1978 AL MAHATA conference was to ensure access to quality health care at lower cost for the entire population.

Despite all the efforts made by ministerial departments and the provincial health inspectorate through its pharmacy office department to make pharmacies open to the public credible and viable, there is still much to be done to improve the management of medicines and medical consumables.

We therefore need to act in line with our detailed recommendations, while insisting on the training and viability of pharmacies open to the public.

Optimizing processes is an important tool, as is training providers in drug management and rational drug prescribing.

It should also be noted that drugs spread out in jars and at the mercy of the population, stored in conditions incompatible with their preservation, inappropriate self-medication of antibacterials widely practiced by patients, substandard, counterfeit or substandard products handled by staff 97% incapable of assessing the quality, safety and efficacy of drugs, are key factors in the rise in morbidity and mortality rates. Consequently, establishments offering substandard and dubious pharmaceutical services are a danger to the emergence of antibacterial resistance. On the other hand, between 20% and 50% of antibiotics are used in agriculture and not in humans; 40-80% of antimicrobials for veterinary use are of dubious value. In addition, limited access to healthcare, lack of regulation of antimicrobial availability, counterfeit or substandard products, poor storage conditions and inadequate infection control in healthcare facilities are all factors within the healthcare system that contribute to the emergence and spread of resistance.

I. RECOMMENDATIONS AND SUGGESTIONS

At the end of our study, we propose the following suggestions to improve the management system for medicines and medical consumables in pharmacies open to the public:

1. To patients or customers receiving services at pharmacies open to the public:

- ❖ To choose reliable and viable pharmacies for good services
- ❖ Verify the quality of care or services offered by pharmacies before purchasing medicines and medical consumables.
- ❖ Supervise the dosage and prescription of drugs available in pharmacies

1. TO THE GOVERNMENT OF RD CONGO

- ❖ Ensure the construction and establishment of viable and reliable pharmaceutical pharmacies.
- ❖ Raise awareness and sensitize service providers in pharmacies to ensure that patients receive appropriate and correct medical prescriptions;
- ❖ That economic operators who own pharmacies hire pre-qualified personnel, in this case pharmacists, for the relational management of medicines;
- ❖ Recommend to providers the use of manual management and organization of medicines and medical consumables when setting up or opening a pharmaceutical dispensary.

2. TO OWNERS OF PHARMACIES

- ❖ Before setting up or opening a pharmaceutical dispensary open to the public, you need to have the necessary documents in place to ensure the viability and reliability of the structure and to guarantee good service.
- ❖ An organization and management manual for medicines and medical consumables;
- ❖ Direct prescriptions according to patients' health problems;
- ❖ To be systematically retrained in pharmacy for a good dispensing of services in pharmaceutical officers;
- ❖ To source medicines and medical consumables from reliable and viable certified wholesalers;
- ❖ Wearing a smock at all times;
- ❖ The use of all materials and documentation essential for proper medication management;

BIBLIOGRAPHY

1. Aida S., Articles sur la pénurie de médicament dans l'Union Européenne : Les causes et les solutions, 2020, P.2-3;
2. Albert T., Problématique de la prise en charge des médicaments essentiels de la liste officielle du Mali par les établissements d'importation et de vente en Gros des produits pharmaceutiques, 2021, P.11 ;
3. Alexandre B., la gestion des stocks des médicaux au sein des pharmacies hospitalières, Analyse des difficultés rencontrées au sein d'hôpitaux généraux en Wallonie, 2022, P.8-20
4. Annie H. and Marie A., Manuel de gestion de la pharmacie dans les centers de santé au niveau périphériques 2016 , P.3-15;
5. Antoine M., Managing drugs and medical devices in hospitals, 2019, P.10-21;
6. Article on essential medicines, 2020, P. 20;
7. Boudjemai T., la gestion des médicaments en milieu hospitalier, cas du Chu de Tizi-Ouzou, 2017,P.13-24 ;
8. Dr. Ernold J., The Great Deadly Epidemics, 2023, P. 27 ;
9. Dr. Peyrand, L'accessibilité des soins de santé en RDC, 2020, P.2;
10. Fidèle M., La circulation des médicaments dans la sphère de la santé, 2020, P.3-6;
11. Fredéric D., Le marché des médicaments, un défi de la couverture universelle de santé, 2022, P.10 ;
12. Grawitz, Méthode des sciences sociales, ed. DALLOZ, PUF, Paris 1982, P.15-20 ;
13. Isabelle G., Pharmacy networks in the United States, 2018, P.12 ;
14. Kikuni S., Gestion des médicaments et matériels médicaux dans la zone de santé des Bagira/Kasha. Cas de HGR de Bagira, 2015 , P.2-6 ;
15. Kwete M., Gestion et approvisionnement en médicament essentiel, 2029, P.39-43 ;
16. La Rousse, 2019;
17. M. Benjilali, l'analyse de la gestion de médicaments et dispositifs médicaux au niveau de la pharmacie hospitalière ces du Chp de Fes (Algha isani), 2021, P.35- 49;
18. Manya K., L'utilisation des soins de santé de base facteurs favorisant la qualité de santé, 2023, P.2-5;
19. Marie-Christine B. and Alain A., Rapport de l'académie nationale de pharmacie sur l'industrialisation des médicaments, 2018, P.2-7 ;
20. Marie-Parile K., Private sector and pharmaceutical industry in Africa, 2018, P.4 ;

21. Médecin sans frontières, organization and management of a pharmacy, 2017, P.2-16;
22. Medication management training module, Min. Santé 4, 2016, P. 24;
23. SSP management training module at ECZ P.6, 2022, P. 6;
24. Module on Introduction to medical equipment management, WHO technical series on medical devices, P.4, 2015;
25. Module tout savoir sur l'officine de pharmacie, 2018, P.1-10;
26. NICOLE S., addressing shortages of médicine, April 2020, P.12 ;
27. S. Zambara, WHO report on access to essential medicines, 2014, P.13 ;
28. S. Zambara, WHO World Health Report, 2010, P.7 ;
29. Tedros A., WHO Essential Medicines, 2018, P.14-15 ;
30. Thomas et All, Production et accessibilité des médicaments en Afrique le secteur privé en principe actif, 2019, P. 4-12 ;
31. Tim E. and Wim Van L., The World Health Report, 2018, P.17 ;
32. Yohane K., L'approvisionnement des médicaments dans les ménages de la zone de santé de Kadutu 2015, P.7-15;
33. Zaina J., Counterfeit medicines kill 270,000 people per in the Sahel, 2023, P.1-5 ;

APPENDIC

SURVEY QUESTIONNAIRE

We are a researcher. We are conducting a survey on "*The management of medicines and medical consumables in pharmaceutical dispensaries open to the public in the Ibanda Health Zone*". Thank you for agreeing to contribute to this survey by answering the questions below.

I. SOCIO-DEMOGRAPHIC CHARACTERISTICS

1. Sex: a) Mb) F
2. Age range: a) 18-22 years b) 23-28 years c) 29-34 years d) 40 years and over
3. Marital status: a) Single b) Married c) Widowed e) Divorced
4. Level of education: a) none b) primary c) secondary d) university
5. Religion: a) Catholic b) Protestant c) Muslim d) Kimbanguist e) Jehovah's Witness f) Other to specify...
6. Profile: a) Pharmacist b) Nurse c) Healthcare professional d) Doctor e) Without
   f) others to be specified:..

II. QUESTIONS IN THEIR OWN RIGHT

7. How long has the pharmacy been in operation?
   a) 0 - 1y b) 2 - 5y c) 6- 10y d) > 10y

8. What operating documents do you have?

a) Notice o f location b) Minutes of contract c) Opening authorization d o c u m e n t

d) without

9. Where does your operating manual come from?

a) IPS b) DPS c) commune d) mairie e) other...

10. What is your source of drugs?

a) CDR b) Hospitals c) Wholesale d) Donation e) Import

11. Do you have a drug and consumable management manual?

a) Yes b) No

12. How do you deliver medicines and medical consumables?

a) a) by medical prescription b) by customer explanation c) after test or consultation

Thank you!

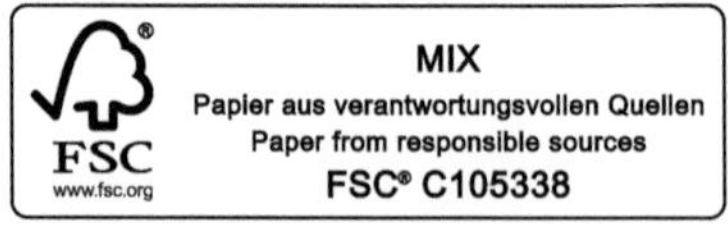

Printed by Books on Demand GmbH, Norderstedt / Germany